KITSCHY ARCHETYPES & REAL DEITIES

a Satanic guide for addiction recovery

THIS BOOK IS WRITTEN FROM MY PERSONAL
PERSPECTIVE BASED ON MY EXPERIENCE AS
A RECOVERING ALCOHOLIC/ADDICT

I DO NOT SPEAK FOR ANY REHAB OR RECOVERY PROGRAM

I AM NOT QUALIFIED NOR I DO DESIRE TO
GIVE MEDICAL ADVICE.....THIS SHOULD COME
FROM A LICENSED PROFESSIONAL WHO KNOWS
YOU AND YOUR MEDICAL HISTORY

(and even then I'd suggest you ask questions and ask what
all of your options are for treatment of any kind)

DEDICATION

This book is dedicated to Satan, Hecate, Santisima
Muerte, Ganesha and to Satanists in recovery

ABOUT ME……

I am an Spiritual Satanist who has been clean and sober
for 9 years. I first got sober through AA in Philadelphia,
Pennsylvania in 2001 as a practicing Pagan. My sponsors
were all Atheists who gave me a simple practical
understanding and usage of the 12 step program.

I went on to sponsor others and served on service commitees in
AA and helped form a CMA (Crystal Meth Anonymous) meeting.

I stayed sober and clean for 6 consecutive years…..later
moved to New Hope, Pennsylvania where I relapsed.

Eventually, I wanted to get sober again but had no
desire to attend AA meetings as the Christian paradigm
had become too distasteful to me since 'converting' to
Satanism in 2010…..even with an Atheistic approach.

So I began searching online for recovery groups for
those who practice 'alternative' religions. All I could
find were Pagan groups…..which was not a problem as
I had practiced Wicca for 13 years previously.

I joined one, participated a lot..had a meaningful experience for
awhile, but the RHP (Right Hand Path) perspective wasn't really
gelling with my developing LHP (Left Hand Path) perspective.

So, I started a group of my own…..an LHP recovery page
on facebook for Satanists (Atheistic, Theistic, etc.),
Luciferians, practitioners of Thelema, Santeria, Chaos
Magic, etc……and have since joined other recovery
groups on facebook that resonate with me.

I have been clean and sober now ..for 9
years with only online support.

2

FOREWORD...

My reason for writing this book is that all too often folks who don't honor a biblical god are told that there is no other way to recover. This simply isn't true. I've stayed sober without this belief.....I know Atheists, Pagans, Buddhists, Satanists, Thelemites, etc.....who've not only gotten clean and sober, but who also maintain continuous long term sobriety.

THIS MAIN BODY OF THIS BOOK INCLUDES 4 SEPARATE SECTIONS............EACH INCLUDES A CORRESPONDING: SEASON, ELEMENT, KITSCHY ARCHETYPE, AFFIRMATIONS, KITSCHY CIRCLE CASTING, AND A MEDITATION WITH A REAL DEITY.....DESIGNED TO AID YOU IN RECOVERY AS A SATANIST

FALL - YOUR THOUGHTS HELP SHAPE YOUR REALITY

1 STORYBOOK WITCH - is often depicted as having green skin and unpleasant facial features, wearing all black, donning a pointed hat and riding a household broom.

FOR OUR PURPOSES - Her element is AIR which relates to the MIND / INTELLECT / UNCONSCIOUS / PSYCHOLOGY.

The deity associated with her is Hecate in Her Crone aspect. She is the Greek goddess of the Underworld, Death, and aids those who have passed on.

AFFIRMATIONS

I WILL BATTLE ONE ADDICTION AT A TIME, (or as many that threaten my immediate well being)

ONE DAY AT A TIME,

IF NECESSARY - ONE HOUR AT A TIME,

BUT I WILL NEVER TRY TO TAKE ON TOO MANY CHALLENGES AT ONCE

AND ALLOW MYSELF TO BECOME OVERWHELMED.

THE EUPHORIC 'PINK CLOUD' PHASE IN MY RECOVERY PROCESS IS A TASTE OF GOOD THINGS TO COME

BUT I WILL NOT MISTAKE IT FOR AN EXCUSE TO BECOME COMPLACENT

I WILL RECOGNIZE AND ALTER MY THINKING WHEN I

FALL INTO OLD NEGATIVE PATTERNS THAT ENCOURAGE
ME TO SEEK OUT MY DRUG/BEHAVIOR OF CHOICE

I WILL FIND AND USE HEALTHY SANE
MATURE WAYS TO DEAL WITH STRESS

RATHER THAN FALLING INTO ADDICTION OR
ADDICT THINKING AS SUBSTITUTES FOR
DESIRABLE COPING MECHANISMS

CAST A (KITSCHY) CIRCLE.......in whichever direction you like

(EACH QUARTER'S CHARACTER CAN BE REPRESENTED
BY......A TOY, A PHOTO, ORIGINAL ART, ETC)

then, call the quarters..........starting in The East

- "STORYBOOK WITCH representing the EAST and the
element of AIR......I ask that you bring wisdom to this
space"........(wait until you feel the presence of the AIR
element)......" You are here, Hail and Welcome"

- "DAPPER DEVIL representing the SOUTH and the
element of FIRE ....I ask that you bring passion to
this space"......(wait until you feel the presence of the
FIRE element)......"You are here, Hail and Welcome"

- "EGYPTIAN MUMMY representing the WEST and the element of WATER ......I ask that you bring serenity to this space".........(wait until you feel the presence of the WATER element)......"You are here, Hail and Welcome"

- "LUCKY LEPRECHAUN representing the NORTH and the element of EARTH......I ask that you bring confidence to this space"......(wait until you feel the presence of the EARTH element)......"You are here, Hail and Welcome"

LIGHT A CANDLE (in the color of your choice) in honor of Hecate

MEDITATION

CLOSE YOUR EYES and imagine a beautiful sunny Fall day..........the air is crisp and slightly chilly. You are walking in a wooded area along a well trodden path.... the leaves of many colors are blowing in the wind and falling to the ground................ You wander off the path to do some exploring and find yourself walking in mud just outside the entrance to an underground cave.

KNOCK THREE TIMES on the old wooden door at the entrance to the cave.........wait until you hear keys rattling and the door will gently creak open.

ENTER....... give your eyes a moment to adjust as the cave is illuminated only by candles.

YOU SEE Hecate seated at a throne.........ask Her how you may better use the power of your mind to aid in your recovery and success....(I'll leave the rest of the Meditation to you)

..........(She may give you something to take with you) when you are through talking to Hecate, respectfully offer thanks. ....Leave the way you came in, closing the door behind you.

Find your way back to the path.........then back to your starting point.......OPEN YOUR EYES.

EXTINGUISH the candle.

RESPECTFULLY RELEASE THE QUARTERS.....

beginning in The North.......

- "LUCKY LEPRECHAUN representing the NORTH and the element of EARTH......I thank you for aiding me and for attending my rite" ......(wait until you feel Him depart)......"You are gone, Hail and Farewell"

- "EGYPTIAN MUMMY representing the WEST and the element of WATER ......I thank you for aiding me and for attending my rite" ....(wait until you feel Her depart)....."You are gone, Hail and Farewell"

- "DAPPER DEVIL representing the SOUTH and the element of FIRE ....I thank you for aiding me and for attending my rite"......(wait until you feel Him depart)....."You are gone, Hail and Farewell"

- "STORYBOOK WITCH representing the EAST and

the element of AIR......I thank you for aiding me and for attending my rite" ....(wait until you feel Her depart)......"You are gone, Hail and Farewell"

TAKE DOWN THE CIRCLE in the direction opposite to that which it was cast.

FINIS

SUMMER - PASSION AND POWER CAN
BE WEILDED RESPONSIBLY.

2 - DAPPER DEVIL - is often depicted as being very well groomed and with pleasing facial features. He is often dressed in a stylish man's suit, with a necktie and freshly shined shoes. His demeanor is one of quiet control with a great ability to stay focused.

FOR OUR PURPOSES: His element is FIRE which relates to the EGO and to MAGIC.

The deity associated with Him is SATAN. He is of many mythologies and goes by many names, but always fosters individual fortitude and endurance in His devotees and admirers.

AFFIRMATIONS

I RECOGNIZE THAT WILL POWER ALONE

DOES NOT ALTER UNCONSCIOUS THOUGHT
PATTERNS AND ADDICTIONS

AND THAT I MUST GO DEEPER TO
EFFECT MEANINGFUL CHANGE

I WILL USE HONESTY AS A TOOL TO AID IN MY
RECOVERY AND IN OBTAINING SELF KNOWLEDGE

I KNOW THAT MAINTAINING SOBRIETY WITHOUT
CONTINUAL PROGRESS ISN'T ENOUGH TO SATISFY
MY HEALTHY EGO AND SENSE OF PRIDE

I ACCEPT RESPONSIBILITY FOR THE CORRECTION OF
ANY OF MY UNDESIRED FLAWS, IMPERFECTIONS,
POOR DECISIONS, ETC.......EVEN IF THEY ARE
NOT ENTIRELY SELF - CREATED

CAST A (KITSCHY) CIRCLE.......in whichever direction you like

(EACH QUARTER'S CHARACTER CAN BE REPRESENTED BY......A TOY, A PHOTO, ORIGINAL ART, ETC)

then, call the quarters..........starting in The South

- "DAPPER DEVIL representing the SOUTH and the element of FIRE ....I ask that you bring passion to this space"......(wait until you feel the presence of the FIRE element)......"You are here, Hail and Welcome"

- "EGYPTIAN MUMMY representing the WEST and the element of WATER ......I ask that you bring serenity to this space"........(wait until you feel the presence of the WATER element)......"You are here, Hail and Welcome"

- "LUCKY LEPRECHAUN representing the NORTH and the element of EARTH......I ask that you bring confidence to this space"......(wait until you feel the presence of the EARTH element)......"You are here, Hail and Welcome"

- "STORYBOOK WITCH representing the EAST and the element of AIR......I ask that you bring wisdom to this space"........(wait until you feel the presence of the AIR element)......" You are here, Hail and Welcome"

LIGHT ONE RED CANDLE AND ONE BLACK CANDLE in honor of Satan.

MEDITATION

CLOSE YOUR EYES...it's a hot Summer night, but with a cool breeze. You return home after a busy day out in the world......open your front door, to an empty room.........a gorgeously ornate armoire appears before you. You find the key that opens it tied around your neck on a red string. You unlock the doors and swing them both open.

Next, you look through the very attractive selection of men's suits and choose the one you'd like to wear (regardless of your gender or gender identity). You put it on along with a beautiful pair of black shiny shoes (whatever style you like - men's dress shoes, high heels, etc)

On your left there is an antique floor length mirror and a dresser. The dresser's surface is stocked with accessories, cosmetics, colognes, perfumes, etc.

Admire yourself in the mirror while you fix your hair, put on cologne, apply cosmetics, etc........take your time......relax and enjoy the way you feel, smell and look.

When you are satisfied....

OPEN YOUR EYES...

TAKE A MOMENT TO 'CHILL'...

keep your eyes open

When you feel ready.....remain still and focus on your actual image in a mirror, relax your mind......and fix your gaze...............watch as your features change, the lighting in the room changes.....you may see different gods, goddesses and daemons in your reflection as the changes occur.

CLOSE YOUR EYES....

When you feel ready....say "Satan, please hear me" - He will make His presence known in a way which is meaningful to you personally. Ask Him how you can better use your personal strengths to aid in your recovery and in your Life..........allow images, thoughts, etc to fill your mind without judging them or trying to control them.......just go with it.

When you are through, offer respect and gratitude to Satan for taking the time to share with you.

OPEN YOUR EYES

EXTINGUISH the candles.

RESPECTFULLY RELEASE THE QUARTERS.....

beginning in The EAST.......

- "STORYBOOK WITCH representing the EAST and the element of AIR.......I thank you for aiding me and for attending my rite" ....(wait until you feel Her depart)......"You are gone, Hail and Farewell"

- "LUCKY LEPRECHAUN representing the NORTH and the element of EARTH.......I thank you for aiding me and for attending my rite" ......(wait until you feel Him depart)......"You are gone, Hail and Farewell"

- "EGYPTIAN MUMMY representing the WEST and the element of WATER ......I thank you for aiding me and for attending my rite" ....(wait until you feel Her depart)....."You are gone, Hail and Farewell"

- "DAPPER DEVIL representing the SOUTH and the element of FIRE ....I thank you for aiding me and for attending my rite"......(wait until you feel Him depart)....."You are gone, Hail and Farewell"

TAKE DOWN THE CIRCLE in the direction opposite to that which it was cast.

FINIS

WINTER - CHANGE CAN BE DIFFICULT TO ACCEPT BUT IS WELL WORTH THE EFFORT

3 EGYPTIAN MUMMY - is usually depicted as being wrapped from head to toe in dingy white bandages. Little else is exposed 'cept her eyes. She is often quite mysterious and sometimes violent.

FOR OUR PURPOSES: Her element is WATER which relates to the EMOTIONS and to SPIRIT.

The deity associated with Her is SANTISIMA MUERTE. She

is the Aztec / Mexican goddess of the Underworld. She is a
favored much by LGBT folks and other marginalized groups.
She does not judge your motives but blindly responds to
requests if She is approached respectfully and lovingly.

AFFIRMATIONS

I KNOW IT'S OK TO BE UNCOMFORTABLE
SOMETIMES IF REACHING MY GOAL REQUIRES
IT AND IT CAUSES ME NO TRUE HARM

EMOTIONAL MATURITY MAY ELUDE ME AT TIMES
BUT IT IS WHAT I STRIVE TO ACHIEVE

I EMBRACE MY ANGER AND ACCEPT RESPONSIBILITY
FOR IT'S EXPRESSION AND MANIFESTATION

IF I NEVER LEAVE MY COMFORT ZONE I WILL WITHER
AND DIE..... OR AT LEAST DIE OF BOREDOM

CAST A (KITSCHY) CIRCLE.......in whichever direction you like

(EACH QUARTER'S CHARACTER CAN BE REPRESENTED
BY......A TOY, A PHOTO, ORIGINAL ART, ETC)

then, call the quarters..........starting in The West

- "EGYPTIAN MUMMY representing the WEST and the
element of WATER ......I ask that you bring serenity to
this space"........(wait until you feel the presence of the
WATER element)......"You are here, Hail and Welcome"

- "DAPPER DEVIL representing the SOUTH and the
element of FIRE ....I ask that you bring passion to
this space"......(wait until you feel the presence of the
FIRE element)......"You are here, Hail and Welcome"

- "STORYBOOK WITCH representing the EAST and the
element of AIR......I ask that you bring wisdom to this
space"........(wait until you feel the presence of the AIR
element)......" You are here, Hail and Welcome"

- "LUCKY LEPRECHAUN representing the NORTH and
the element of EARTH......I ask that you bring confidence
to this space"......(wait until you feel the presence of the
EARTH element)......"You are here, Hail and Welcome"

LIGHT A CANDLE to honor Santisima Muerte. (white
for healing, black for banishing, red for obtaining)

MEDITATION

CLOSE YOUR EYES It's a beautiful Winter evening,
the air seems fresh and clean and snowflakes are
gently falling to the ground around you.

The streets are dimly lit but you see an old storefront with
a seemingly warm glow at it's entrance off in the distance.

You decide to take a closer look and begin walking
toward it. The ground is slippery at times as there
are icy patches beneath the fallen snow so you must
proceed carefully and not lose your footing.

You arrive at the storefront and peer into the window. You
realize that the glow is created by the fire burning inside. You
see an old woman seated in a rocking chair, in front of the
fireplace with Her back to you. She is gently rocking back
and forth as she knits a garment of white (or black, or red)

You knock on the door.

Without turning around, she gestures for you to come inside.

There is a wooden chair to her left with a small table beside it.

As you are sitting you remember the chocolates and tobacco you
have been carrying around with you. You know She would truly
appreciate them so you place them on the table as a gift for Her.

Thank Her for inviting you in and tell Her of your
need or desire. (I'll leave the rest to you).

When you are through, offer respect and gratitude to
Santisima Muerte for taking the time to hear you, and
remind Her that you have left gifts for Her as you exit.

Make your way through the accumulated
snowfall back to your starting point.

OPEN YOUR EYES

EXTINGUISH the candle.

RESPECTFULLY RELEASE THE QUARTERS.....

beginning in The North.......

- "LUCKY LEPRECHAUN representing the NORTH and
the element of EARTH......I thank you for aiding me
and for attending my rite" ......(wait until you feel Him
depart)......"You are gone, Hail and Farewell"

- "STORYBOOK WITCH representing the EAST and
the element of AIR......I thank you for aiding me and

for attending my rite" ....(wait until you feel Her depart)......"You are gone, Hail and Farewell"

- "DAPPER DEVIL representing the SOUTH and the element of FIRE ....I thank you for aiding me and for attending my rite"......(wait until you feel Him depart)....."You are gone, Hail and Farewell"

- "EGYPTIAN MUMMY representing the WEST and the element of WATER ......I thank you for aiding me and for attending my rite" ....(wait until you feel Her depart)....."You are gone, Hail and Farewell"

TAKE DOWN THE CIRCLE in the direction opposite to that which it was cast.

FINIS

SPRING - I WILL CREATE AND NURTURE THE LIFE I DESIRE

4 LUCKY LEPRECHAUN - is usually depicted as a jovial spry gnome donning green garments and holding a pot of gold coins. He might grant wishes but is possessive of his own property.

FOR OUR PURPOSES: His element is EARTH which relates to the BODY and to SCIENCE.

The deity associated with Him is GANESHA. He is the Hindu god of abundance, earthly pleasure, and the remover of obstacles. He can be prayed to to clear one's mind of distractions.

AFFIRMATIONS

I KNOW THAT 'WHITE KNUCKLING' THROUGH CHALLENGING TIMES IN SOBRIETY IS A TEMPORARY SOLUTION AT BEST

AND I CAN DO BETTER FOR MYSELF

MY LIFE IS MORE MEANINGFUL AND ENJOYABLE TO ME WHEN I SEEK WAYS TO GROW AND IMPROVE

TRADING ONE ADDICTION FOR ANOTHER DOES NOT EQUAL SUCCESS

I WANT MORE OUT OF LIFE

I EXERCISE MY BODY AND MY MIND

I WANT TO BE THE BEST VERSION OF ME

CAST A (KITSCHY) CIRCLE.......in whichever direction you like

(EACH QUARTER'S CHARACTER CAN BE REPRESENTED
BY......A TOY, A PHOTO, ORIGINAL ART, ETC)

then, call the quarters..........starting in The NORTH

- "LUCKY LEPRECHAUN representing the NORTH and
the element of EARTH......I ask that you bring confidence
to this space"......(wait until you feel the presence of the
EARTH element)......"You are here, Hail and Welcome"

- "STORYBOOK WITCH representing the EAST and the
element of AIR......I ask that you bring wisdom to this
space"........(wait until you feel the presence of the AIR
element)......" You are here, Hail and Welcome"

- "DAPPER DEVIL representing the SOUTH and the
element of FIRE ....I ask that you bring passion to
this space"......(wait until you feel the presence of the
FIRE element)......"You are here, Hail and Welcome"

- "EGYPTIAN MUMMY representing the WEST and the
element of WATER ......I ask that you bring serenity to
this space"........(wait until you feel the presence of the

WATER element)......"You are here, Hail and Welcome"

LIGHT A CANDLE (a color that inspires joy
in you) to honor GANESHA

MEDITATION

CLOSE YOUR EYES..... It's a chilly Spring morning-
you are slightly uncomfortable as you begin your
day ......'cause you're wearing only a t-shirt and shorts
but choose to keep going rather than return home.

You make your way to a toepath in a wooded area
and start jogging. Your body temperature begins
to rise and your heart rate increases.

You feel the Sun on your skin,

the aroma of Nature's bounty is all around you.....you
breathe it in as you continue on the toepath.

You feel grateful to be alive.

Off in the distance you catch a glimpse of brightly
colored fabrics blowing in the breeze.

You start slowing down a little ....then stop, catch your
breath ......and begin walking at a relaxed pace. You veer
off the toepath and walk towards the beautiful colors.

As you get closer you begin to hear a slow steady
drum beat (that will continue throughout
your visit)........you keep walking.

You reach your destination......and find the, elephant
headed god, GANESHA seated on a bright red cusion
with a small pond before Him, a single large bright
pink lotus flower rests on the water's surface.

He sees you........and gestures for you to sit beside Him on
the bright blue cushion to his right. Ask Him how you can
more effectively create the change you'd like to see in your
Life. (I'll leave the rest of the meditation to you).....

.....When you are through He hands you an object
that will remind you of the advice He has given
you.......... offer Love and gratitude to GANESHA.

You leave..... find your way back to the toepath.......and
begin jogging back to your starting point.

You reach your home.

OPEN YOUR EYES

EXTINGUISH the candle.

RESPECTFULLY RELEASE THE QUARTERS.....

beginning in The WEST.......

- "EGYPTIAN MUMMY representing the WEST and the element of WATER ......I thank you for aiding me and for attending my rite" ....(wait until you feel Her depart)....."You are gone, Hail and Farewell"

- "DAPPER DEVIL representing the SOUTH and the element of FIRE ....I thank you for aiding me and for attending my rite"......(wait until you feel Him depart)....."You are gone, Hail and Farewell"

- "STORYBOOK WITCH representing the EAST and the element of AIR......I thank you for aiding me and for attending my rite" ....(wait until you feel Her depart)......"You are gone, Hail and Farewell"

- "LUCKY LEPRECHAUN representing the NORTH and the element of EARTH......I thank you for aiding me and for attending my rite" ......(wait until you feel Him depart)......"You are gone, Hail and Farewell"

TAKE DOWN THE CIRCLE in the direction opposite to that which it was cast.

FINIS

COMMON TOPICS IN RECOVERY PROGRAMS

RELAPSE......

this is a subject that comes up a lot in recovery. Rehabs and other programs tell us that relapse is a part of recovery. While it is a part of some of our 'stories'......you do not have to relapse on your recovery 'journey'.....it is not a given. If one does relapse, of course, this does not have to end his/her/their recovery.

EGO......

is talked about so often in recovery programs and in many spiritual belief systems. The most common belief is that ego is 'bad'...it has to be shrunken down or gotten rid of

entirely.

The Ego is necessary for survival....without it we would have no reason to work...as we wouldn't desire anything. We might not even feed ourselves.....as this requires a 'selfish' desire.

Arrogance and false pride are not the same as Ego......these interfere with any chance we have for true success in recovery as they take us further away from the truth about ourselves......our strengths and weaknesses.

HUMILITY....

It is important to be teachable. If we approach recovery with obstinance we have little chance for success....as with learning any new skill a reasonably open mind can be truly beneficial.

INTROSPECTION......

A lot of recovery programs will ask us to reflect on the past....our addiction-it's consequences, how it effected us, our lives, and those around us. This is not to be taken lightly as it's an important reminder of what we don't want to repeat.

MOTIVATION......

I learned through AA that it's important for me to do the 'right' thing regardless of what motivates me. I don't have to be filled with love and selflessness in order to do a 'good' deed or to help another. I can do it solely to benefit my recovery.

RECOVERY PROGRAMS.....

There are 12 step programs, AA Agnostica, SMART Recovery, Rational Recovery, rehab, Inpatient, Intensive Outpatient.......just to name a few. Recovery programs can be very helpful, especially, if you don't know where to start.

WORKING A PROGRAM.....

If you're going to bother to participate in a recovery program it makes sense to get all you can out of it. Just showing up and watching the clock.....waiting for the meeting or session to end isn't likely to benefit you. If a program is absolutely not working for you try a different one.

SPONSORSHIP.....

Should you decide to work a 12 step program.....it will most likely be suggested to you that you get a sponsor. A sponsor's primary function is to teach you the 12 steps and help you 'work' them.......this requires more than just reading about them. The sponsor is not designated to try to convince you of or dissuade you from any beliefs or belief system......if you find yourself in this kind of sponsor-sponsee relationship...move on to a different sponsor. You don't necessarily have to share the same beliefs or lack of belief, but it works best if this is left to personal choice for each of us.

Once you find a sponsor who you want to work with......the relationship works best as a teacher-student kind of relationship.....you being the student.

PEER SUPPORT......

I find this to be invaluable. It is so important to effectively communicate with other recovering folks. It helps us feel less isolated and less unrealistically unique. Connecting with others really enhances sobriety and our sense of well being and it can even be enjoyable.

PRAYER.......

This, of course, can be beneficial to those with some sort of 'Higher Power'...whether it's a pantheon, god/goddess, devil, demon, angel, inner guide.........whatever.

It's a chance to quiet the mind and connect with a being/concept that we trust to guide us in the 'right' direction.

AFFIRMATIONS.....

Anyone can use them....and if your totally opposed to prayer it's a great option to help shift your focus from 'negative' thought patterns and self destructive behaviors. They don't have to be cheezy.....they should be meaningful to you.

MEDITATION....

Much of the time meditation eludes me, but I do find reading and playing video games for reasonable amounts of time meditative.

Paying attention to your breathing and letting your thoughts go can be a fine method of meditating.

FORGIVENESS......

This is discussed to help one let go of the past. It is considered to be a gift we give ourselves. Of course it's not always a reasonable reaction to unreasonable people or situations.......but for small matters it can be very helpful.

TURNING IT OVER......

'Turning over' your problems to another or to others can be great for reducing stress and for finding solutions to problems we can't make sense of. If one has a 'Higher Power'

the request for a solution can be made. If one is Atheist/
Agnostic.....asking your peers for their input might be helpful.

SELF CARE.......

When in active addiction many of us, myself included,
didn't take proper care of ourselves or our true needs.
As recovering folks we generally become healthier
and develop healthier habits. This includes our;
physical, mental, and for some....spiritual lives.

TOOLS......

Recovery programs offer 'tools' to help us along our
'journey'. These can include ideas for.....relapse prevention,
stress management, coping with our emotions, etc.

TRIGGERS.....

Recovery programs generally encourage us to avoid
temptation, especially in early recovery.

We may want to stay away from people and places that afford
easy access to the substance/behavior we wish to eliminate.

PERSONAL RESPONSIBILITY.....

Emotional immaturity is common among addicts and the
tendency to blame others for our problems.....seriously. In
recovery we start to learn that not only is our recovery our
responsibility....our lives, decisions, and choices are too.

MEDICATIONS...

Advice about medications should always come from a
professional..in a professional setting. If a doctor doesn't seem
to be helping you... don't be afraid to get a second opinion.

Self medicating, whether the stuff is legal or not,
is not likely to be beneficial for recovery.

While others in recovery can share their personal experience
with medications with you....this should not be taken as sound

medical advice for you personally. We don't all respond to medications the same nor have identical medical histories.

SERVICE....

It is often recommended to help new people in recovery as well as yourself. This is not only a really decent thing to do...but it really does help our own recovery. One valuable benefit is that it reminds us what early recovery was like and why we don't want to go back to living as an addict.

GRATITUDE......

Being grateful for what you do have....what you value.....material objects, those you love-human, animal, divine, etc....is not only logical, but it's a great way to eliminate mild depression and self pity.

MORALS....

These are to be determined by the individual as long as we're not infringing upon the rights of others.......which is just really shitty.......we have every right and the responsibility to determine these for ourselves.

THE 7 DEADLY SINS.......

Our natural desires are not 'bad' or 'evil'. We do, however, benefit from coping with them wisely. While humans are a species of animal....we are not feral.

WRATH.....

While anger is a healthy normal reaction to some of life's challenges ....how we handle it can be important. I know I can't carry around a mind full of anger and lead an enjoyable productive existence. Expressing anger is important..but the more sane and rational the method the better.

SLOTH....

It's important to get adequate rest. Having trouble getting a good night's sleep in early recovery is not uncommon........look for healthy ways to unwind and calm yourself at the end of the day....if you can't sleep just try to relax your mind.

GREED....

The desire for more than you have right now is a sign of a well person with healthy desires......just don't let wanting more keep you from enjoying and appreciating what you do have...it's foolish.

LUST.....

Lust is completely natural and extremely powerful at times. We will know what fulfills our natural desires in the most personally beneficial ways better than anyone else.....and what enhances our sobriety.

Masturbation is often recommended, especially for early recovery, as it releases tension and helps keep us from making poor relationship choices.

Stating new 'romantic' relationships in early recovery is often frowned upon as it is a time when we benefit more from focusing on ourselves.

ENVY....

Envy can be a great motivator. When someone has something I want ....I can feel inspired to work to get it for myself as well.

As long as I don't use it to feel sorry for myself or to resent others for what they have worked for (or have been given- none of my business really) it can be truly beneficial.

GLUTTONY......

Gluttony can easily be compared to an addiction as it implies irrational over indulgence. Anything done in excess becomes unhealthy and actually, unenjoyable.

Wanting more is healthy but should be tempered with wisdom and self respect.

VANITY......

There's nothing wrong with feeling good about yourself....proud of your accomplishments....pleased with your appearance, but it's also important to appreciate the efforts of others which have benefited you.

WHAT I FIND USEFUL......

STOICISM...

Stoicism is concerned with accepting what is, what has happened.....and being grateful for our experiences.

It encourages us to accept responsibility for our thoughts, actions and behavior.

JUNG.....

Carl Jung's writings are very useful for anyone who wants to explore his/her/their inner world.......what motivates them, what hinders them, personal 'demons', etc.

He was also a great influence for the formation of the AA program.

OCCULT PRACTICES....

I use ritual, spell work, the Tarot, and the study of occult material to aid in my recovery and in all aspects of my life.

Ritual, whether viewed as 'real' or as a purely psychological exercise....can help focus the mind and release 'negative' emotions.

Spell work can be used to let go of what no longer serves us......unhealthy habits, attachments, etc.

The Tarot can be used when seeking solutions to problems or psychologically as a mirror of human behavior and the many parts of the 'psyche'.

Study not only gets me 'out of my head', but it also helps me formulate new ideas and appreciate the wisdom of authors I admire.

THE BASIC REQUIREMENTS FOR RECOVERY....

DESIRE....

The true desire to get out of the addiction.....if it's not something you want for yourself it's not likely recovery will work for you at the present time.

DO IT FOR YOU.....

Getting clean/sober for someone else doesn't seem to be very effective....do it for you...and others will benefit as well.

CHANGE.....

You are likely to experience many changes in your life and in yourself as you recover. Don't let this scare you to the point where you give up....if you truly want to recover. Talk about it, reach out.....you don't have to everything alone.......and you can always return the favor.

AFTERWORD.....

Anyone who truly wants to get sober/clean can....regardless of- age, race, sexual orientation, gender identification, economic status, occupation, belief, lack of belief, cultural background, past behavior, incarceration, etc...

Just as addiction does not discriminate...neither does the recovery process.

Whatever method or methods you choose for your recovery.....all the best and much success to you.

LHP (suggested) 16 steps of recovery

DAVID RIVERA·MONDAY, FEBRUARY 6, 2017·

step 1....I accepted that I cannot control my
alcoholism/addiction alone

step 2....came to the realization that I
need help to get sober/clean

step 3....made the decision to ask for and accept
help.. getting and living sober/clean

step 4....took an inventory of my behaviors and decisions
that I disliked or did not benefit me when drinking/using

step 5....shared this list with another. (sponsor,
therapist, counselor, deity, etc..)

step 6....prepared to take action to change
my thought/action process

step 7....took action to change my thought/
action/decision making process. (meditation,
ritual, therapy, rehab, meetings, etc..)

step 8....made a list of relationships,
property, etc. that I damaged.

step 9...took action to take responsibility for my actions and
to set things 'right'. (paying for damaged property, etc./
behaving like a' better' brother, sister, father, mother, etc.)

step 10..strived to remain mindful of my behaviors and

decisions that I disliked or did not benefit me now, sober/clean
(possible examples: people pleasing, mooching, laziness, etc..)

STEP 11...CONTINUED TO TAKE ACTION TO CONTROL/CHOOSE MY BEHAVIOR THROUGH MEDITATION/RITUAL/THERAPY/OTHER

STEP 12..SHARED MY (RECOVERY) EXPERIENCE WITH OTHERS...IT MIGHT HELP THEM AND IT WILL STRENGTHEN MY RECOVERY AND SOBRIETY

step 13...no longer carried RESENTMENTS {poison to an alcoholic}, cursed, forgave, resolved, etc....dealt with the anger and moved on.

step 14...did not let myself get too BORED {time bomb for an addict}, a bored addict will want to use eventually.

step 15...gave up my drinking buddies, junkie friends, old hangouts, etc.. if I can't remain clean and sober when I revisit these people and places.

step 16...continued to ask for and offer help where and when it benefits me,(my recovery) and, when willing, (the recovery of) others.